OK KETO,
I SEE YOU

OK KETO, I SEE YOU

Akimmy Nedina Wheeler

To order additional copies of this book, contact:
Xlibris
844-714-8691
www.Xlibris.com
Orders@Xlibris.com
833989

Contents

Keto Meal Recipes

Fast Food

Whether you think you can, or
think you can't, you're right.

—Henry Ford

Disclaimer

Hey, guys, I just want to say—surprise, I'm not a doctor. Bummer, I know. I've never been in the healthcare field. Well, I did take a few phlebotomy classes. I did not complete the course, however. I shouldn't have ever started them. I don't even like needles! Anyway, it was a different time. I was in a different place. Yadda-yadda-yadda. Moving on. I do want you to know that the information provided throughout this book pertaining to your health or wellness, exercise, relationships, or any other aspect of your life does not create a dietitian-patient relationship and is not intended to be a substitute for professional medical advice, diagnosis, or treatment.

The information that I have presented is intended for informational purposes only.

Who Am I?

Who am I? Not the girls dem sugar. OK, sorry, that was a horrible Beenie Man joke. I know.

I'm an interior designer that practices as a BIM/CAD technician, a part-time domestic violence advocate, and a part-time sales associate at a department store. In my spare time, I volunteer with AmeriCorps, my local recycling center, and Bridging the Gap.

When I began my journey with keto, my focus wasn't on losing weight. I'm busy! I'm too busy to diet, too busy to exercise, too busy to think about losing weight!

At the time, I was working in an excessively-toxic workspace. I was in the midst of a friendship breakup. Those hurt the most! COVID had just hit. My eldest sister who has asthma caught COVID from her job. My car was broken into. People I knew were losing their jobs left and right.

My part-time job furloughed everyone. And my apartment flooded. I had to move out of my apartment for a week. And it happened to start snowing.

If anything could have described my situation, it would have been the opening lyrics from "Gravity," a song from John Mayer's *Continuum* album: Gravity is working against me, and gravity wants to bring me down . . .

I had gotten my foot stuck in the train tracks, metaphorically speaking, as the speeding train of life blared behind me. It showed absolutely no signs of stopping.

For the first time in a long time, I did not have control over my life nor my situation. I needed to somehow bring back my control. I needed something that would help me find my control or just a *control*.

J. P. Morgan said, "The first step towards getting somewhere is to decide that you are not going to stay where you are."

The first step for me was finding a routine. I could control a routine. I knew that I needed to start there. Keto was my routine.

While on the keto diet, I lost a total of 130 pounds in ten months, and I was able to eliminate and pinpoint the toxic relationships and habits within my life.

As I've mentioned before, I'm a busy person, but I was able to curate a version of the keto diet that matches my lifestyle. I found quick and easy recipes, snacks, a workout plan, and a very easy-breezy routine.

I hope this book can help do the same for you.

Keto: How It works
and How I Use It

Without sounding too scientific, keto is an eating pattern that works by activating ketone molecules in your blood. It is a diet that advocates for low-carb, high-fat foods, with a moderate amount of protein.

Still confused? Well, here is another explanation: It's a diet that involves your metabolism to switch from glycolysis (sugar-burning) to ketosis (fat-burning).

This is why carbs and sugar are restricted on this diet. This has especially been hard for a carbatarian like me.

I was and am an excessive snacker! I've never wanted full meals. I've simply wanted food to accompany whatever activity that I was doing at the time. Party snacks.

Without thinking about it, I'd have excessive amounts of chips and dip, scones, cookies (the good fresh-baked kind!), Lord-only-knows-how-much pasta! Don't get me started on sweets! When I ate sweets, *I ate sweets!* Do you hear me?!

My food relationship, of course, was created after a routine that I inadvertently fell into.

I was a busy college student with two jobs, I had no time to focus on healthy food. Much like other college students, my diet consisted of quick and microwavable food.

This routine and habit, of course, followed me after graduation into the work field. I was a starving young professional who would work late hours and early morning. Sometimes I'd work from 8:00 AM one day until 3:00 AM the next day.

Fast food was definitely a huge part of my life and routine. My social circle religiously went to restaurants at least twice a week. Myself included!

On the Border and McDonald's were some of the common favorites.

After work, for two years, I would go to McDonald's and order three fresh cookies, sometimes six in a single sitting! Yes, six!

Each cookie holds a total of 170 calories, 15 grams of sugar, and 22 grams of carbs.

An order of three cookies would fetch you 510 calories, 45 grams of sugar, and 66 grams of carbs.

An order of six cookies would fetch you 1,020 calories, 90 grams of sugar, and 132 grams of carbs.

The dietary guidelines for Americans recommend that carbs make up 45–65 percent of your daily calorie intake. On a recommended 2,000 calorie daily intake, between 225 and 325 carbs should be eaten per day; 66–132 grams of carbs were used on cookies alone!

Hold on, reader, what we are not going to do is act like those fresh, hot, and soft cookies from McDonald's that ooze with melted semi-sweet chocolate chips are not addictive!

I had to say that for those of you who were about to fix their mouths to say something negative about my ex-routine habit. Judge your, mammy, not me! Moving on. I would eat the cookies on top of whatever else that I ate for breakfast, lunch, dinner, and night snacks.

I enjoyed my relationship with everyday foods, but it too had to come to an end.

My relationship and its routine.

The first step for you is to figure out what type of relationship you have with food.

You don't have to write it down, just take a mental note. Your life and routines are different from mine. My journey and your journey through keto will be different.

Not everyone eats because they're sad, because they're depressed, because they're bored. Dude, food is just good sometimes! I get it!

I don't know your reasoning, but you do.

Your first step, your first aim at keto, is going to be you figuring out where is your "problem area" when it comes to food. Do you go bananas over sweets? Do you eat for boredom? Are you a social eater, you eat when you're in activity with others?

Help yourself by starting with the type of eater that you are and what are your eating routine patterns.

Within this book, there are meal plans and suggestions for snacks. You don't have to follow them. These are merely suggestions.

The key is to work with yourself, not against it.

What to Expect When Starting the Keto Diet

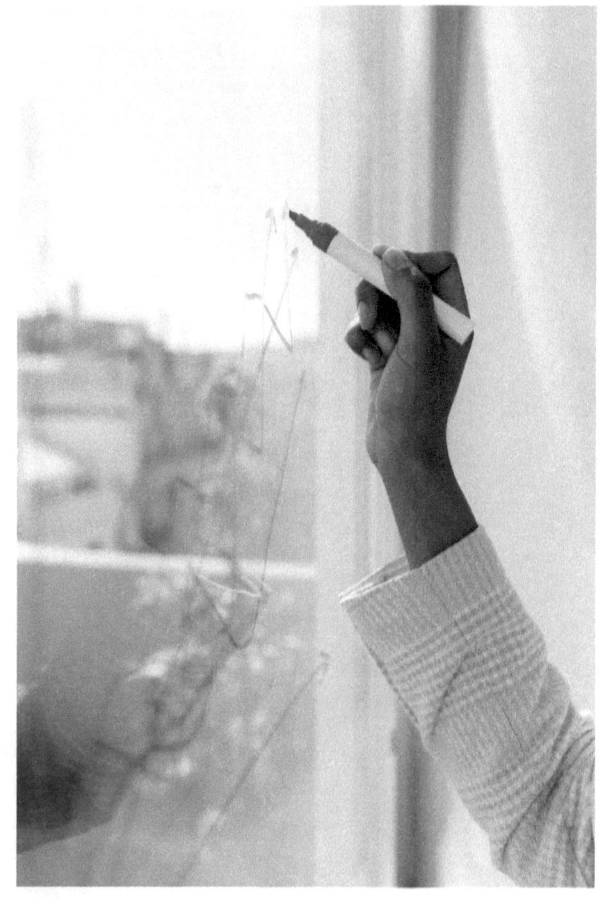

KETOSIS TIMELINE

12–24 HOURS	*KETONES BEGAN TO BE PRODUCED*
*4–5 DAYS**	*KETO FLU SYMPTOMS KICK IN*
1 WEEK	*WEIGHT LOSS SHOULD BEGIN*
2 WEEKS	*DECREASED HUNGER, MORE ENERGY*
4 WEEKS	*DECREASED INSULIN*

* Healthline.com says it takes typically two to four days to enter into ketosis. It took me three days to start experiencing the keto flu.

– Everyone is different, it may take some longer than others to enter ketosis. There is nothing wrong with it, do not get discouraged. Try eating 20g of carbs or lower to enter into ketosis much faster.

* Keto Flu symptoms include: headaches, fatigue, nausea, and increased thirst. (I had horrendous headaches on the third day of my keto journey, on the fourth day they subsided).

KETOGENIC DIET

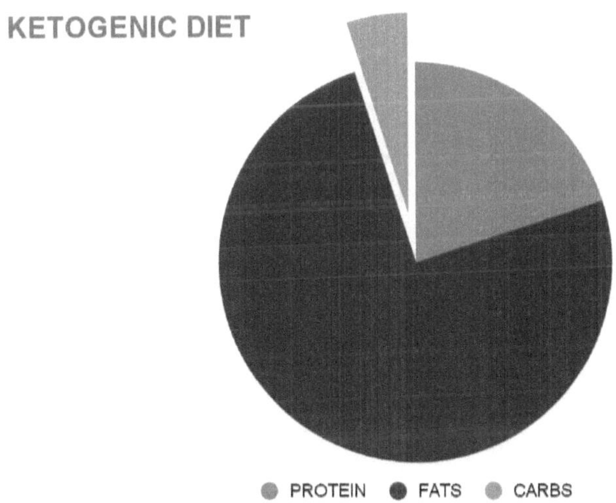

You should have a diet made up of 5 percent carbs, 70 percent fats, and 20 percent protein.

Do's and Don'ts of Keto: What to Eat and What Not to Eat

You don't have to eat everything on this list. Stick to what you like! This is your keto journey, not anyone else's—period.

VEGGIES

Artichokes
Asparagus
Broccoli
Brussel sprouts
Cabbage
Cauliflower
Celery
Cucumber
Garlic
Green beans
Kale
Kimchi
Leeks
Lettuce
Mushrooms
Okra
Onions
Peppers
Pumpkin
Sauerkraut
Spinach
Sugar Snap Peas
Tomatoes
Zucchini

DRINKS

All teas
Broth
Coffee
Lemon & lime juice
Water

MEAT

Bacon
Beef
Bison
Chicken
Cured meats
Duck
Goat
Lamb
Organ meats
Pork
Poultry
Rabbit
Steak
Turkey
Veal
Venison

NUTS & SEEDS

Almonds
Brazil nuts
Hazelnuts
Macadamia nuts
Pecans
Pine nuts
Walnuts
Flaxseed
Hemp seeds
Pumpkin seeds
Sesame seeds
Sunflower seeds

FATS

Avocado oil
Beef tallow
Butter
Cocoa butter
Coconut butter
Duck fat
Extra virgin olive oil
Ghee
Goose fat
Lard
Macadamia oil
MCT

DAIRY

*No low fat
*No fat-free

Do's and Don'ts of Keto: What to Eat and What Not to Eat

<u>FRUIT</u>

Avocado
Berries
Coconut
Lime
Lemon
Olives
Rhubarb

<u>FLOUR</u>

Almond flour
Coconut flour
Other nut flour
Psyllium flour

<u>EGGS</u>

Any how you prefer

<u>FISH & SHELLFISH</u>

Cod
Crab
Halibut
Lobster
Mackerel
Mussels
Oysters
Plaice
Salmon
Sardines
Scallops
Shrimp
Trout
Tuna

<u>OK ARTIFICIAL SWEETNERS</u>

Brazzein
Curculin
Erythritol
Glycerol
Glycyrrhizin
Inulin
Isomalt
Lactitol
Luo han guo
Mannitol
Miraculin
Natural sweetener
Oligofructose
Sorbitol
Sugar alcohol
Sugar fiber
Xylitol

<u>NOT OK ARTIFICIAL SWEETNEERS</u>

Agave syrup
Aspartame
Brown rice syrup
Caramel
Dextrose
Fructose
Galactose
Gold syrup
HFCS-42/
HFCS-55/
HFCS-90
Lactose
Maltodextrin
Maltose
Maple syrup
Neotame
Sucralose
Sucrose
Trehalose

Helpful Gadgets and Tools During Keto

No, you don't have to have everything on this list. However, they will help make your keto journey go by much smoother. If you can't do all these, please make it your business to own serving-size bowls and measuring cups.

- Silicone baking mats
- Muffin pans
- Baking pan with lid
- Food scale
- Ziploc bags (at least two different sizes to store food in)
- Pyrex (or any plastic container sets)
- Body/weight scale
- Measuring cups
- Cup bowls/serving size bowls
- Calendar/planner
- Strainer
- Keurig/Coffee pot
- Whisk

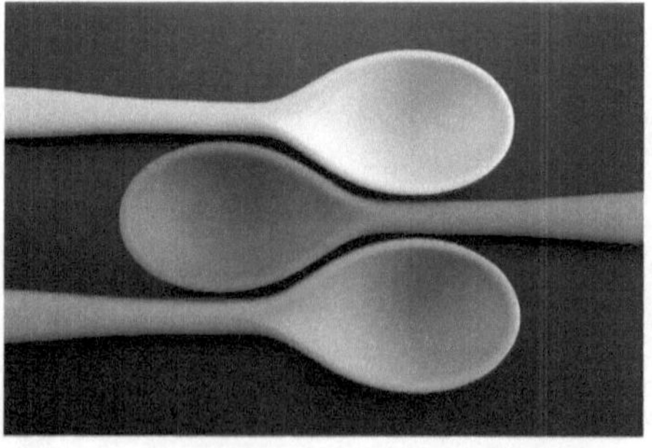

Essential Food Items

These are food items that I purchased for my keto recipes more times than not. Each of the listed items are very affordable and will save you time when cooking the recipes.

- Two to three different varieties of cheese (ex. cheddar, Colby jack, mozzarella)
- Cauliflower
- John Soules Foods brand fully-cooked rotisserie seasoned chicken
- John Soules Foods brand fully-cooked oven-roasted chicken
- John Soules Foods brand fully-cooked grilled chicken
- John Soules Foods brand fully-cooked beef steaks
- Great Value brand thick-cut naturally-hickory-smoked cooked bacon
- Cauliflower rice
- Zucchini noodles
- Squash spaghetti
- Nasoya Pasta Zero spaghetti-shaped shirataki
- Accent seasoning
- Slap Ya Mama seasoning
- Heavy whipped cream
- Scallions/green onions
- Stevia/sugar substitute

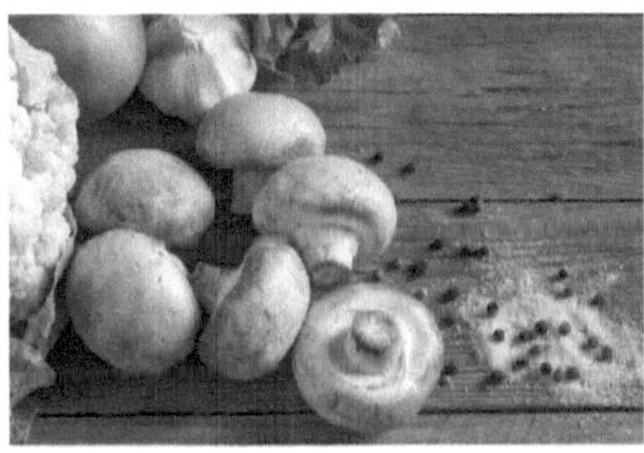

KETO MEAL RECIPES

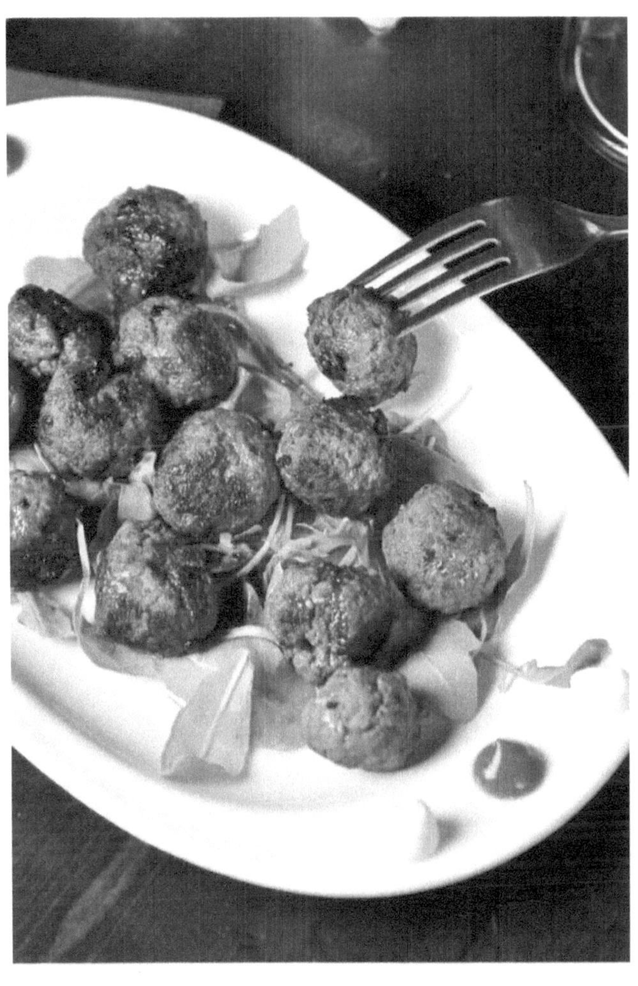

Keto Burger

Ingredients:

- 1 1/4 lbs. ground beef or ground turkey
- 1 1/4 teaspoon Accent seasoning
- 2 teaspoon seasoning salt
- 1 teaspoon ground black pepper
- 2 teaspoon Slap Ya Mama
- 1 teaspoon oregano
- 1 teaspoon garlic powder
- 1/3 cup red onion, finely chopped
- 1 fresh bell pepper, cut into small pieces
- 1 pack fully-cooked bacon
- 1 1/4 cup avocados, cut lengthwise
- 1 1/4 butter or romaine lettuce
- 10 slices Colby jack cheese
- 16 oz. sliced baby bella mushrooms

Instructions:

Preheat the oven to 425°F.

Line a baking sheet with parchment paper and set it aside.

Add the ground beef, seasoned salt, black pepper, oregano, Slap Ya Mama, garlic powder, bell pepper, and onions to a bowl and mix to combine.

Form into 5–6 patties and place on the prepared baking sheet.

Bake in a preheated oven for 18 minutes (or until your liking).

Brown the bacon a bit to extract some of the grease to fry the mushrooms. Once the bacon is brown, remove it from the pan and place the mushrooms in the grease. Cook the mushrooms

for 5–6 minutes. You're looking for a brown color. Once done, remove from fire.

Remove the baking sheet from the oven, top the burgers with cheese and return to the oven.

Bake for 1–2 more minutes.

To serve, spread on a serving of avocado onto the lettuce leaves and top with mushrooms and a serving of bacon. Serve immediately.

I always freestyle my burgers, and you can as well. Remember to read the label and ingredients. A good BBQ sauce is from the G Hughes SmokeHouse brand. It's sugar-free and does not hold many carbs. Whatever you do, keep in mind your carb intake.

Serving 5, calories 530, carbohydrates 4 g.

Loaded Cauliflower Casserole

Ingredients:

2 14.4 oz bags of frozen cauliflower florets
1 box (8 oz.) cream cheese softened
1/2 cup sour cream
1 1/2 cups sharp cheddar, finely shredded
1 1/2 cups Monterey Jack cheese, finely shredded
1 teaspoon garlic powder
1/2 teaspoon onion powder
1 pack of pre-cooked bacon slices
1/4 cup chopped fresh chives (reserve 1 tablespoon for the top)
Salt and pepper to taste
1 teaspoon Accent seasoning

Instructions:

Follow instructions on the bag of cauliflower florets (until fork tender); approximately 5 minutes. Drain well in a colander.

Preheat the oven to 425 degrees. Grease 9 x 13-inch baking dish.

In a large bowl, combine cream cheese, sour cream, cheddar cheese, Monterey Jack, garlic powder, Accent seasoning, and onion powder. Mix until creamy and smooth. Gently stir in the cauliflower, 1/2 of the bacon, and chives. Season with salt and pepper to taste.

Spoon into the casserole dish and top with remaining bacon. Bake uncovered for 20–25 minutes or until the cheese is melted. Top with remaining chives and serve.

This recipe was one of my very first keto recipes, and I must say that it is a meal that I would eat off the keto diet as well. Be careful with your seasonings on this recipe, don't overdo it with the salt. Keep in mind that cheese is salty. This will appear to affect your water weight on the scale.

Serves 12, calories 276, total carbohydrates 6.3 g.

Buffalo Chicken and Cauliflower Casserole

Ingredients:

1 14.4 oz. bag of frozen cauliflower florets
4 oz. cream cheese
1 8 oz. bag John Soules Foods rotisserie-style chicken breast strips
2 cloves garlic, crushed
1/2 cup RedHot buffalo wings sauce
3 tablespoons heavy cream
4 oz. cheddar cheese, shredded
1 tablespoon Accent seasoning

Instructions:

Preheat the oven to 400°F. Then microwave the cauliflower, follow the instructions on the bag (until fork tender); approximately 5 minutes. Drain well in a colander.

Add the cream cheese, hot sauce, Accent seasoning, and garlic to a skillet. Whisk and when the cream cheese has melted, add in the chicken and cauliflower. Mix well and take off the stove.

Spray a 9 x 13-inch baking dish and spoon the mixture in. Pour the heavy cream over the top and then sprinkle the cheddar cheese.

Place the pan into the oven and bake for about 30 minutes or until it's nice and browned on top.

Garnish with green onions.

This recipe gave me life! Before eating this, I had never eaten a buffalo cheese dip nor sauce.

This was my introduction to the buffalo sauce world, and, honey, I'm glad to be here.

Serving 4, calories 390, total carbohydrates 3 g net.

Taco Lettuce Wraps

Ingredients:

1 2/3 lbs. ground beef or turkey
1/4 cup onion, finely diced
2 cloves garlic
2 packets taco seasoning
2/3 cup water
1/4 cup salsa
1 head iceberg lettuce or butter lettuce

Toppings as desired, such as freshly-grated cheese (Monterey Jack or extra-sharp cheddar), olives, thinly-sliced avocado or guacamole, sour cream, jalapenos, freshly-chopped cilantro, chopped cherry tomatoes, etc.

10–12 firm large pieces of lettuce

Instructions:

Wash and gently separate lettuce leaves. Place in the refrigerator.

Brown beef, onion, and garlic until no pink remains. Drain fat.

Stir in taco seasoning, water, and salsa. Bring to a boil, reduce to a simmer and cook until thickened.

Cool for 5 minutes.

Spoon meat mixture into lettuce cups and top with toppings as desired.

Optional toppings: pico de gallo, avocado, sour cream, cheese

Try using parchment paper with this recipe to help with the mess. Serving 4, calories 307, carbohydrates 4 g.

Meatloaf and Mashed Cauliflower

Ingredients:

1 tablespoon olive oil
1/2 small onion, diced
2 cloves garlic, minced
1 2/3 lbs. lean ground beef
2 teaspoon Italian seasoning
1/2 teaspoon salt
1/4 teaspoon pepper
1 teaspoon Accent seasoning
1 teaspoon seasoning salt
2 tablespoons fresh parsley
1 green bell pepper, diced
2 large eggs
1/4 cup shredded parmesan cheese
1/4 cup almond flour

Topping:

1/3 cup of sugar-free ketchup
2 12 oz. bags Birds Eye brand sour cream
chives
mashed cauliflower
1/2 stick of butter

Instructions:

Preheat the oven to 400°F. Line a small pan with foil and spray with cooking spray.

Cook onion and garlic in olive oil until tender. Cool completely.

Combine all meatloaf ingredients in a bowl and mix well.

Form into a 3 x 8-inch loaf and place on a prepared pan.

Bake for 30 minutes uncovered. Top with topping and bake an additional 30–40 minutes or until loaf reaches 160°F (or until no longer pink in the middle).

Rest for 5–10 minutes prior to serving.

Follow instructions on mashed Cauliflower bags. Once cooked, combine both bags, mix in butter, salt, and pepper for taste.

Serve with meatloaf.

Loaf: Serving 5, calories 239, carbohydrates 6 g.
Mashed cauliflower: Serving 5, calories 45, carbohydrates 5 g net.

Cauliflower Cheeseburger Casserole

Ingredients:

- 1 lbs. ground meat
- 2 14.4 bags cauliflower florets
- 2 teaspoon steak seasoning
- 1 teaspoon Accent seasoning
- 1 teaspoon onion powder
- 1 pack cheesy taco seasoning
- 1/4 cheddar cheese, shredded
- 1/2 cup Colby jack, shredded
- 1 tablespoon butter, melted
- 4 oz. cream cheese, cut into cubes
- 2 eggs
- 1/2 cup heavy cream
- 1/2 cup cheddar cheese, shredded

Instructions:

Preheat the oven to 400°F.

Follow the instructions on the bag (until fork tender); approximately 5 minutes.

In the meantime, add the beef to a skillet and sprinkle steak seasonings, Accent seasoning, and onion powder on top.

Once brown, drain meat.

Sprinkle in cheesy taco seasoning.

In a medium pot, add cauliflower, cream cheese, and 1/4 cup of cheddar cheese.

Mix well and then pour into the baking dish. Add meat, and mix well.

In a bowl, beat eggs then whisk in cream and butter.

Pour over beef mixture and top with remaining 1/2 cup of cheese.

Bake for 30 minutes.

You can also add a bit of salsa on top, just remember to watch your carbs and calories intake for the day.
Serving 6, calories 421, carbohydrates 2.6 g.

Spaghetti and Meatballs

Ingredients:

2 tablespoons extra-virgin olive oil
3 garlic cloves, crushed
1 large onion, finely diced
1 2/3 lbs. ground beef
2 tablespoons Accent seasoning
1/2 cup shredded parmesan
1 tablespoon dried oregano
2 tablespoons black pepper
1/2 teaspoon salt
1/4 cup beef broth
14 oz. canned diced tomatoes, no added sugar
1 package zucchini noodles or spaghetti squash or shirataki spaghetti
2 tablespoons shredded parmesan per plate
2 tablespoon Italian seasoning
1 large egg

Instructions:

In a bowl, mix the minced beef with ground beef, grated parmesan, egg, dried herbs, and all other seasonings.

Shape meatballs with your hands and form 20 meatballs.

In a large saucepan, under medium heat warm olive oil.

Add the crushed garlic and diced onion, reduce to low heat and cook for 2 minutes until golden and fragrant.

Add the meatballs into the saucepan and fry the meat for 2–3 minutes on all sides.

Add the beef broth to deglaze and stir in the can of diced tomatoes.

Cover and simmer for 20 minutes or until the liquid slightly thickens and reduces.

Adjust with salt and pepper to taste.

Meanwhile, cook the noodles following your packing instructions. If you can't find these noodles you can make your own zucchini noodles with a spiralizer.

When the keto noodles are cooked, serve 1/4 cooked noodles per plate (or more, they have zero carbs so they won't impact carb count, but they will add fiber). Top with 1/4 of the whole meatball sauce.

Try Brazi Bites with this meal, just watch your carb and calorie intake for the day.
Serve with 1/4 cup of grated parmesan.
Serving 4, calories 365, carbohydrates 6.4 g.

Jalapeño Beef Casserole

Ingredients:

1/4 cup heavy cream
1/2 teaspoon onion powder
1/2 teaspoon garlic powder
2 teaspoon Accent seasoning
2 teaspoon seasoning salt
1 pack taco seasoning
2 oz. pepper jack cheese
2 oz. Colby jack cheese
1/4 cup jalapeño, diced, seeded or unseeded, as preferred
4 oz. cream cheese
1 pack of precooked bacon
1 2/3 lbs. ground beef
1 16 oz. sour cream

Instructions:

Preheat oven to 350 degrees.

Combine onion powder, garlic powder, Accent seasoning, and seasoning salt. Mix well and set aside. Seed, if desired, and diced jalapeños and set aside.

Brown the ground beef over medium-high heat, seasoning with a combined spice mixture.

Remove meat from fire and drain. Return to fire and add a packet of taco seasoning.

Once seasoning is completely mixed, lower heat and add heavy cream and cream cheese.

Stir to mix.

Once the cream cheese is melted and smooth, add 2/3 of jalapeños, 1/2 of the bacon, and pepper jack cheese. Mix well.

Transfer the mixture to an 8 x 8-inch pan and top with Colby jack cheese, bacon, and jalapeños.

Place in oven for 5 minutes or until brown and bubbly.

Allow to cool for 5–10 minutes to serve immediately, or cool a little longer before portioning for meal prep.

When serving, add a dollop of sour cream.

I must admit, this meal can be a bit spicy. If need be, only add half of the requested jalapeño amount.
Serving 5, calories 585, carbohydrates 2 g.

Club Lettuce Wrap

Ingredients:

2–3 leaves of iceberg lettuce
2 slices of cheese (Swiss, provolone, cheddar, whatever you prefer)
3 slices of ham
2 slices of bacon, cooked
3–4 small tomato slices or 1 Campari tomato
2 pickle sandwich slices
Mustard, mayo, salt pepper, if desired

Instructions:

Layout a piece of wax or parchment paper.

Lay 2–3 slices of lettuce slightly overlapping.

Top with cheese, ham, bacon, pickles, tomato, mustard, mayo, salt, and pepper, if desired.

Wrap tightly and use the wax or parchment paper to help you keep the wrap secure.

Sandwich wraps are fairly easy and quick meals. Some other honorable-mention wraps are bacon, ham, and egg wrap (calories 330, carbohydrates 7 g); ham, Swiss, and tomato (calories 302, carbohydrates 6.9 g); turkey bacon ranch (calories 472, carbohydrates 5.8 g).

Add in a few cucumbers and, if possible, barbecue sauce! If it is a crunch that you are wanting, try out some parm crisps or other cheese chip brands to add to your wrap.

As always, watch your carbs, calories, and sugar intake.

Serving 1, calories 515, carbohydrates 3.9 g.

Chicken Salad

Ingredients:

Chicken:
3 chicken breasts or 1 bag John Soules Foods grilled chicken
4 tablespoons olive oil
1 teaspoon Accent seasoning
1 teaspoon Slap Ya Mama seasoning
Salt and pepper to taste
Salad:
4 boiled eggs, peeled and chopped
2 4-pack of celery, diced
0.75 oz. dill weed, chopped
1/3 cup yellow mustard
1/2 cup mayonnaise
1/4 cup dill relish
1/2 teaspoon garlic powder
1/2 teaspoon onion powder
Salt and pepper to taste
Romaine lettuce leaves for serving the chicken salad

Instructions:

Season the chicken with Accent and Slap Ya Mama seasoning salt, and then brush the chicken with olive oil.

Follow instructions on the package for preparing the meat.

Once the chicken is finished cooking, remove it and let it cool completely.

Once the chicken is cool, shred the chicken with a fork and place it in a medium-sized bowl.

Add the remainder of the ingredients, not including the romaine lettuce, to the bowl with the chicken, and mix everything together. Adjust the seasonings to your preference, adding more or less.

Fill the romaine lettuce leaves with the chicken salad mixture, and enjoy!

Try adding some fresh cucumbers to the recipe and some Jamaican curry, if you're feeling adventurous.
Serving 5, calories 331, carbohydrates 2 g.

Cauliflower Fried Rice

Ingredients:

1 10 oz. bag riced veggies cauliflower
1 pack fully-cooked bacon
2 large eggs
2 medium scallions, sliced thin
2 tablespoons sesame oil
1 tablespoon fish sauce
1 tablespoon soy sauce
1 teaspoon freshly-ground black pepper
1 teaspoon garlic, minced
1 teaspoon ginger, minced
2 teaspoon Accent seasoning

Instructions:

Follow instructions on veggies riced cauliflower on how to cook it. Transfer the riced cauliflower into a container or cookie sheet. Press all your body weight onto a paper towel sitting on top of the cauliflower. The idea is to drain as much water as possible from it. Chop up 2 stalks of scallions to put into the fried rice. Put the bacon into the pan, we want to cook these until they're extra crispy.

Once the bacon is around this stage, you can remove it from the pan.

Put it onto some paper towels to dry off and crisp up. Keep some of the bacon fat in the pan.

Put the cauliflower over the bacon fat and allow it to cook for a moment. Add your soy sauce and fish sauce to the cauliflower fried rice and mix it well.

Put the cauliflower off to the side and add your sesame oil, scallions, garlic, and ginger.

Allow this to cook for a minute and mix everything together well. You can add your pepper at this point.

Push your cauliflower fried rice off to the side and add your 2 scrambled eggs to the pan.

You want the eggs to get to an omelet consistency, so allow them to cook through before you flip them to cook more.

Once the eggs are cooked, break them up into small pieces and add your bacon.

Stir everything well and serve!

Serving 3, calories 214.33, carbohydrates 5.27 g net.

FAST FOOD

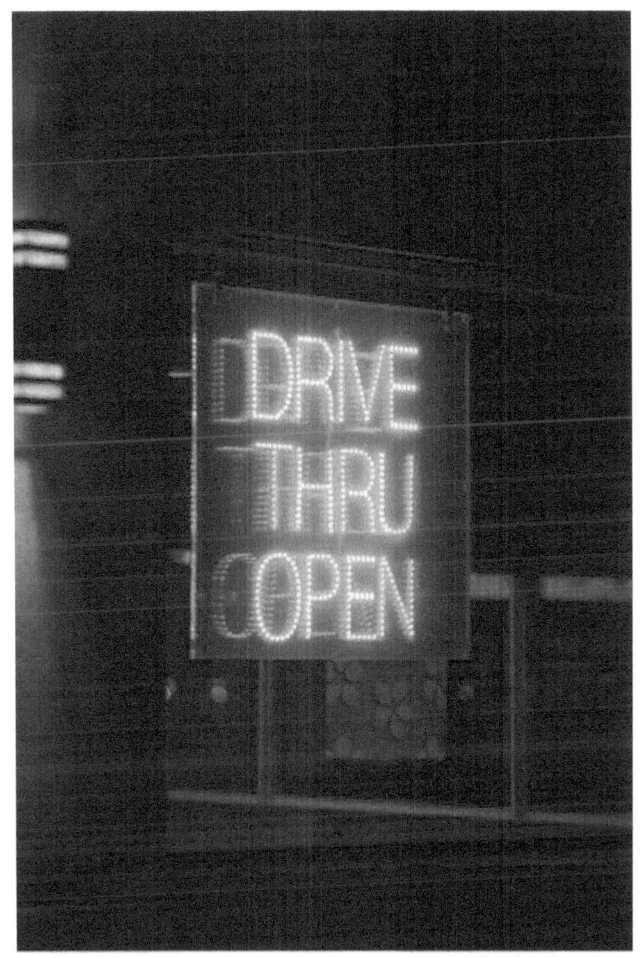

Keto-Approved Burgers (No Buns)

These bunless burgers are keto-friendly and simple fast-food options that will allow you to keep your freedom to eat out. Remember to order simple side salads with high-fat dressings to boost your fiber intake.

Sonic Double Bacon Cheeseburger: 638 calories, 3 g carbs

McDonald's Double Cheeseburger: 270 calories, 4 g carbs

Five Guys Bacon Cheeseburger: 370 calories, 0 g carbs

Wendy's Double Stack Cheeseburger: 260 calories, 1 g carbs

Hardees 1/3 lbs. Thickburger with cheese and bacon: 430 calories, 0 g carbs

Keto-Approved Chicken Sandwiches (No Buns)

Extra mayo has been added to these sandwiches to increase the fat content. When ordering, do make sure that you avoid the sweet sauces (honey, maple, etc.).

Burger King Grilled Chicken Sandwich with extra mayo: 350 calories, 2 g carbs

Chick-Fil-A Grilled Chicken Nuggets dipped in two servings of ranch avocado

dressing: 420 calories, 3 g carbs

Wendy's Grilled Chicken Sandwich with extra mayo: 286 calories, 5 g carbs

McDonald's Pico Guacamole Sandwich: 330 calories, 9 g carbs

Keto-Approved "Unwiches"

These sandwiches have no buns, and even better, you can stick to the "Slims" which are all under 300 calories! (no bread)

Slim 3 (tuna salad): 270 calories, 5 g carbs

The J. J. BLT (bacon, lettuce, tomato, and mayo): 290 calories, 3 g carbs

The Big Italian (salami, ham, provolone, pork, lettuce, tomato, onion, mayo, oil, and vinegar): 560 calories, 9 g carbs

The J. J. Gargantuan (salami, pork, roast beef, turkey, ham, and provolone): 710 calories, 10 g carbs

Keto-Approved Menu Items

These items are actually on the menus as more and more restaurants are taking note of keto's popularity (as they should!).

In-n-Out Burger "Protein Style" Cheeseburger with onions: 330 calories, 11 g carbs

Hardees 1/3 lbs. Low-Carb Thickburger: 470 calories, 9 g carbs

Carl's Jr. Lettuce-Wrapped Thickburger: 420 calories, 8 g carbs

Five Guys Bacon Cheeseburger in a lettuce wrap with mayo: 394 calories, ~1 g carbs

Keto-Approved Burrito Bowls (no rice or beans)

These keto-friendly burrito bowls options are easy to order, simply eliminate the rice and beans. Chipotle has cauliflower rice, if you were in the mood for a rice substitute!

Taco Bell Cantina Power Steak Bowl with extra guacamole: 310 calories, 8 g carbs

Chipotle Chicken Burrito Bowl with cheese, guacamole, and romaine lettuce: 525 calories, 10 g carbs

Chipotle Steak Burrito Bowl with lettuce, salsa, sour cream, and cheese: 400 calories, 6 g carbs

Keto-Approved Salads

It's not uncommon for a salad at any restaurant to be very high in carbs (croutons, tortilla strips, etc.). To keep your salad low in carbs, skip dried fruit, added sugar, and sweet dressings, and breaded meat.

Chipotle Salad Bowl with steak, romaine, cheese, sour cream, and salsa: 405 calories, 7 g carbs

McDonald's Bacon Ranch Grilled Chicken Salad with guacamole: 380 calories, 10 g carbs

Arby's Roast Turkey Farmhouse Salad with buttermilk ranch dressing: 440 calories, 10 g carbs

Snacky Snacks

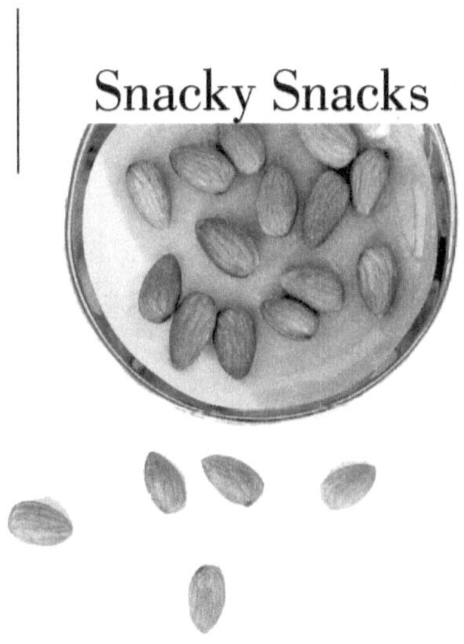

The idea is to have quick pick-ups. Chips, cookies, and other everyday snacks are always easy to obtain, so it only makes sense that I should have quick grabs here and there.

Sweets	Salty	Combinations
Lilly's semisweet chocolate	Oven-roasted almonds	Serving of pepperoni and cheese stick
SlimFast Keto Fat Bombs (caramel chocolate is the best one in my opinion)	Pork rinds: queso flavor, salt and vinegar flavor, salt and pepper flavor, etc.	Great Value snack plate, 3 oz. (choose the one without breadsticks or chocolate)
Simple Mills Brownies, banana bread, pumpkin spice bread	Crazy Richard's Peanut Butter	Jack Link's Meat and Cheese (any meat and cheese sticks)
Keto nut granola trail mix	Quest chips	

As I've mentioned before, I'm a snacker. Snack time is totally a thing for me! Another honorable mention would be Lenny&Larry cookies. Lenny&Larry's peanut butter cookie is the truth! It's not your traditional peanut butter cookie, but it gets the job done. I did not want this list to be overwhelming, I want it to act as a starting place for you. I want this to give you a feel for keto snacks. This is your kindergarten.

As we prepare to move into meal plans and your routine, think about which snack or snacks would be best for you.

*What could be more important than
a little something to eat.*

—*Winnie the Pooh*

Adult Beverages

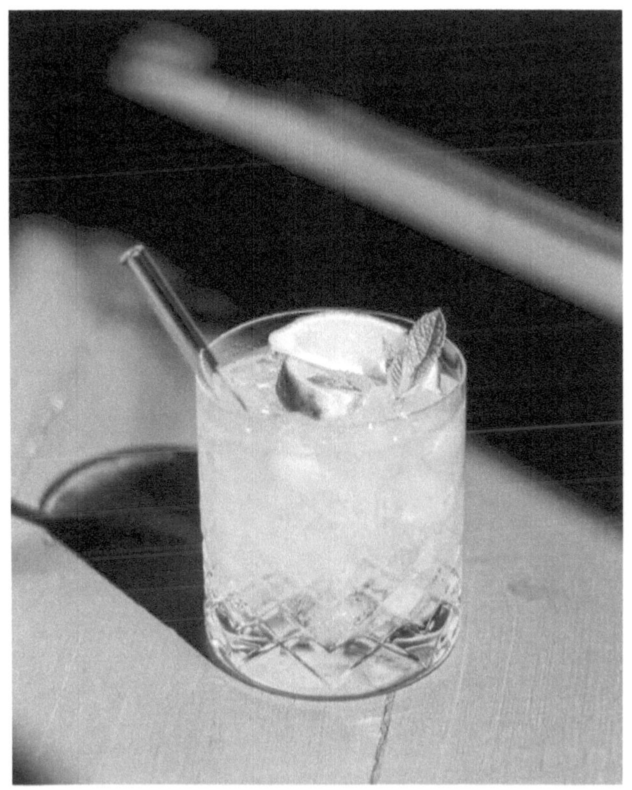

Thank the heavens that there are still plenty of other options for beverages one can enjoy and still remain in ketosis! You can drink alcohol in moderation and simply go with unsweetened alcoholic beverages that are low in carbohydrates.

<u>Alcohols to Drink</u>

Champagne or sparkling wine (90 calories, 2 g net carbs)
Gin (73 calories, 0 g net carbs)
Gin & slimline tonic (148 calories, 7.5 g net carbs)
Red wine (125 calories, 3 g net carbs)
Rum (64 calories, 0 g net carbs)
Tequila (69 calories, 0 g net carbs)
Vodka/Soda (64 calories, 0 g net carbs)
Vodka martini (130 calories, 0 g net carbs)
Whiskey (70 calories, 0 g net carbs)
White wine (120 calories 3 g net carbs)

<u>Mixers</u>

Seltzer/Club soda
Sugar-free tonic water
Unsweetened iced teas
Water

<u>Stay Away from These Mixers</u>

Diet sodas, regular soda
Most beers

<u>Low-to-No-Carb Drinks</u>

Coffee (black or with heavy cream or MCT oil)
Fruit-infused water

High-sugar drinks are likely best to avoid to make sure that one stays in a ketogenic state.

Drinks mixed with juices, frozen drinks, cocktails, and added simple syrups must be avoided.

Do remember that like food, alcohol must not become an abused part of your routine.

Drink because you are happy, but never
because you are miserable.
—G. K. Chesterton

Getting to It

On average, it takes more than two months before a new behavior becomes automatic. The amount of time that it takes for a new habit to form, of course, depends on the behavior, the person, and their circumstances.

The meal plan that I've included in this book is roughly more than two months, it's for ten weeks. I know that everyone isn't perfect, and there will be a day or week that you plateau (weight doesn't go up or down) or gain weight. I feel the ten-week plan will give you confidence during your beginning (or continued) journey in keto.

Things to consider:

- Keep track of times to help you see out your patterns or habits, such as what time you ate, how long you were active, and feelings during those times.
- Remember to work with yourself not against it: Compare your days within the
- ten-week meal plan to learn patterns and become more aware of how you lose weight.
- Figure out which fasting methods would best fit your new routines.
- Start waist training! This helps you form the hourglass shape. (You're welcome.)
- Don't compare anyone else's success with yours! You'll be treading in dangerous waters, my friend.
- It is OK to indulge in junk food! I know that sounds crazy. However, it's to help you stay in ketosis, if that makes sense. For me, this method helped me control my sweet and junk food urges. Just don't go overboard! Example: I enjoy cinnamon-roasted almonds, they're 10 g of carbs per serving, so I cut the serving in half or a third to

cut back on my carb intake for the day. I paired the almonds with something that doesn't have any carbs or extremely low in carbs, like cheese or pepperoni. This is a very dirty keto method.

— You must watch your daily sugar, calorie, and carb intake while doing this. I would not suggest doing this until you've seen how your body reacts to keto. You should wait possibly two weeks after being in ketosis.

My second week of being on my keto diet, I would go to a restaurant called Taste of Philly, and I would order a brat and french fries—yes, french fries. The brat didn't have a bun, and that was my only meal for the entire day. Every Saturday for two months, that was my dirty meal. I did not see a change in the amount of weight that I lost as the meal did not negatively affect my diet.

The only reason I stopped was I got a new job that wouldn't allow for my trip to Taste of Philly to continue.

What I am attempting to say is you can have what you want, you simply must go about it another way. Let's be clear, you can't have your favorite Ben and Jerry's ice cream. However, you can have a substitute from Halo's brand. You can't have your favorite chocolate candy bar, but you can have one of SlimFast's Fat Bombs. You can't have nacho cheese Doritos, but you can have Quest Loaded taco-flavored chips.

There are additional pages, about a week's worth, in this book to help you keep track of your routine and food intake. Should you not be a person to write things down, which is fine, make sure you take good mental notes. Starting out, it is best to study your body and how it reacts to your routine and to keto.

Don't allow this diet to be for naught.

Fasting Methods

The Warrior Fast

Involves the encouragement of subsisting on only small amounts of vegetables and fruit (berries in our case) during the day then eating a single huge meal at night.

The 5:2 Fast

Involves eating 500–600 calories for two days out of the week and eating normally on the other five days.

Alternate Day Fast

Involves fasting every other day, either by not eating anything or by eating only a few hundred calories.

The 16/8 Fast

Involves daily fasting of 16 hours and a restricted 8-hour eating window. During those eight hours, two or more meals will be eaten. When I began my keto journey, I started with this fasting method. On average, I lost 3–3.5 lbs. every week with it. Each day I saw about half of a pound gone on the scale. This was an excellent method for me at the time. However, my work schedule changed, and I knew that I needed to change my fasting method as well.

Eat-Stop-Eat

Involves one or two 24-hour fasts per week. *Should you choose this method, which I currently do, stick to a regular diet as if you hadn't been fasting. I fast on Tuesdays and Thursdays. I don't eat anything on said days, but I do drink water and tea.*

Spontaneous Meal-Skipping

Involves skipping one or two meals when you don't feel hungry or don't have time to eat. *I listed this one to give you knowledgeable options. However, I feel this method could become quite toxic. We are trying to create balanced routines for eating, we are not trying to support broken systems. The broken system, in this case, is "when you don't have time to eat" This idea alone will make you gain weight instead of losing. Remember to fight with yourself, not against it. We are trying to repair your food relationship, not work around it. However, the choice is totally yours.*

Should you feel this is the best method for you, shoot!

Week 1:

Calories per day: 000–1,500
Carbs per day: 0–20 g

Choose your fasting method and apply it to this plan.

* *Freestyles are you choosing from the list of fast foods that are keto-approved.*

Sunday	Monday	Tuesday	Wednesday	Thursday	Friday	Saturday
Meal 1:	Meal 1:	Meal 1:	Meal 1:	Meal 1:	Meal 1:	Meal 1:
2 boiled eggs, serving of Jimmy Dean fully-cooked pork sausage patties, water to drink	2 boiled eggs, your choice of a cheese stick, water to drink	2 boiled eggs, your choice of a cheese stick, water to drink	2 boiled eggs, your choice of a cheese stick, water to drink	2 boiled eggs, your choice of a cheese stick, water to drink	2 boiled eggs, your choice of a cheese stick, water to drink	2 boiled eggs, serving of Jimmy Dean fully-cooked pork sausage patties, water to drink
Meal 2:	Meal 2:	Meal 2:	Meal 2:	Meal 2:	Meal 2:	Meal 2:
Keto burger, keto fat bomb snack, *any keto drink	Keto burger, keto fat bomb snack, *any keto drink	Keto burger, keto fat bomb snack, *any keto drink	Keto burger, keto fat bomb snack, *any keto drink	Keto burger, keto fat bomb snack, *any keto drink	FREESTYLE	FREESTYLE
Snack:	Snack:	Snack:	Snack:	Snack:	Snack:	Snack:
2 keto fat bombs	Great Value snack plate, 3 oz. serving of roasted almonds	Great Value snack plate, 3 oz. serving of roasted almonds	Great Value snack plate, 3 oz. serving of roasted almonds	Great Value snack plate, 3 oz. serving of roasted almonds	2 keto fat bombs	2 keto fat bombs
Cal.: 1,236	Cal.: 1,196	Cal.: 1,196	Cal.: 1196	Cal.: 1,196	*Cal.: 416	*Cal.: 616
Carb.: 12.2	Carb.: 16.2	Carb.: 16.2	Carb.: 16.2	Carb.: 16.2	*Carb.: 5.2	*Carb.: 6.2
						*Keep cal. count

* *Drink your appropriate amount of water! If you're hungry, it's probably because you are actually thirsty. If you choose to drink anything other than water, remember to count your calories and carbs.*

Carbs - Alcohol Sugars - Fiber = Net Carbs

ALL NUTRITIONAL INFORMATION IS APPROXIMATE AND WILL VARY BASED ON ACTUAL INGREDIENTS AND BRANDS USED.

Week 2:

Calories per day: 000–1,500

Carbs per day: 0–20 g

Choose your fasting method and apply it to this plan.

* *Freestyles are you choosing from the list of fast foods that are keto-approved.*

Sunday	Monday	Tuesday	Wednesday	Thursday	Friday	Saturday
Meal 1:	Meal 1:	Meal 1:	Meal 1:	Meal 1:	Meal 1:	Meal 1:
2 boiled eggs, serving of Jimmy Dean fully-cooked pork sausage patties, water to drink	2 boiled eggs, your choice of a cheese stick, water to drink	2 boiled eggs, your choice of a cheese stick, water to drink	2 boiled eggs, your choice of a cheese stick, water to drink	2 boiled eggs, your choice of a cheese stick, water to drink	2 boiled eggs, your choice of a cheese stick, water to drink	2 boiled eggs, serving of Jimmy Dean fully-cooked pork sausage patties, water to drink
Meal 2:	Meal 2:	Meal 2:	Meal 2:	Meal 2:	Meal 2:	Meal 2:
Buffalo chicken and cauliflower casserole, keto fat bomb snack, *any keto drink	Buffalo chicken and cauliflower casserole, keto fat bomb snack, *any keto drink	Buffalo chicken and cauliflower casserole, keto fat bomb snack, *any keto drink	Buffalo chicken and cauliflower casserole, keto fat bomb snack, *any keto drink	Buffalo chicken and cauliflower casserole, keto fat bomb snack, *any keto drink	FREESTYLE	FREESTYLE
Snack:	Snack:	Snack:	Snack:	Snack:	Snack:	Snack:
2 keto fat bombs	Serving of pepperoni, Colby jack cheese stick, serving of roasted almonds	Serving of pepperoni, Colby jack cheese stick, serving of roasted almonds	Serving of pepperoni, Colby jack cheese stick, serving of roasted almonds	Serving of pepperoni, Colby jack cheese stick, serving of roasted almonds	2 keto fat bombs	2 keto fat bombs
Cal.: 1,096	Cal.: 1,024	Cal.: 1,024	Cal.: 1,024	Cal.: 1,024	*Cal.: 416	*Cal.: 616
Carb.: 11.2	Carb.: 12.2	Carb.: 12.2	Carb.: 12.2	Carb.: 12.2	*Carb.: 5.2	*Carb.: 6.2
						*Keep cal. count

* *Drink your appropriate amount of water! If you're hungry, it's probably because you are actually thirsty. If you choose to drink anything other than water, remember to count your calories and carbs.*

Carbs - Alcohol Sugars - Fiber = Net Carbs

ALL NUTRITIONAL INFORMATION IS APPROXIMATE AND WILL VARY BASED ON ACTUAL INGREDIENTS AND BRANDS USED.

Week 3:

Calories per day: 000–1,500
Carbs per day: 0–20 g

Choose your fasting method and apply it to this plan.

* *Freestyles are you choosing from the list of fast foods that are keto-approved.*

Sunday	Monday	Tuesday	Wednesday	Thursday	Friday	Saturday
Meal 1:	Meal 1:	Meal 1:	Meal 1:	Meal 1:	Meal 1:	Meal 1:
2 boiled eggs, serving of Jimmy Dean fully-cooked pork sausage patties, water to drink	2 boiled eggs, your choice of a cheese stick, water to drink	2 boiled eggs, your choice of a cheese stick, water to drink	2 boiled eggs, your choice of a cheese stick, water to drink	2 boiled eggs, your choice of a cheese stick, water to drink	2 boiled eggs, your choice of a cheese stick, water to drink	2 boiled eggs, serving of Jimmy Dean fully-cooked pork sausage patties, water to drink
Meal 2:	Meal 2:	Meal 2:	Meal 2:	Meal 2:	Meal 2:	Meal 2:
Taco lettuce wrap, 2 keto fat bomb snack, *any keto drink	Taco lettuce wrap, 2 keto fat bomb snack, *any keto drink	Taco lettuce wrap, 2 keto fat bomb snack, *any keto drink	Taco lettuce wrap, 2 keto fat bomb snack, *any keto drink	Taco lettuce wrap, 2 keto fat bomb snack, *any keto drink	FREESTYLE	FREESTYLE
Snack:	Snack:	Snack:	Snack:	Snack:	Snack:	Snack:
2 keto fat bombs	Birch Benders Brand Brownie, Crazy Richard's peanut butter	Birch Benders Brand Brownie, Crazy Richard's peanut butter	Birch Benders Brand Brownie, Crazy Richard's peanut butter	Birch Benders Brand Brownie, Crazy Richard's peanut butter	2 keto fat bombs	2 keto fat bombs
Cal.: 1,013	Cal.: 931	Cal.: 931	Cal.: 931	Cal.: 931	*Cal.: 416	*Cal.: 616
Carb.: 12.2	Carb.: 15.2	Carb.: 15.2	Carb.: 15.2	Carb.: 15.2	*Carb.: 5.2	*Carb.: 6.2
						*Keep cal. count

* *Drink your appropriate amount of water! If you're hungry, it's probably because you are actually thirsty. If you choose to drink anything other than water, remember to count your calories and carbs.*

Carbs - Alcohol Sugars - Fiber = Net Carbs

ALL NUTRITIONAL INFORMATION IS APPROXIMATE AND WILL VARY BASED ON ACTUAL INGREDIENTS AND BRANDS USED.

Week 4:

Calories per day: 000–1,500
Carbs per day: 0–20 g

Choose your fasting method and apply it to this plan.

* *Freestyles are you choosing from the list of fast foods that are keto-approved.*

Sunday	Monday	Tuesday	Wednesday	Thursday	Friday	Saturday
Meal 1:	Meal 1:	Meal 1:	Meal 1:	Meal 1:	Meal 1:	Meal 1:
2 boiled eggs, serving of Jimmy Dean fully-cooked pork sausage patties, water to drink	2 boiled eggs, your choice of a checse stick, water to drink	2 boiled eggs, your choice of a cheese stick, water to drink	2 boiled eggs, your choice of a cheese stick, water to drink	2 boiled eggs, your choice of a cheese stick, water to drink	2 boiled eggs, your choice of a cheese stick, water to drink	2 boiled eggs, serving of Jimmy Dean fully-cooked pork sausage patties, water to drink
Meal 2:	Meal 2:	Meal 2:	Meal 2:	Meal 2:	Meal 2:	Meal 2:
Loaded cauliflower casserole, keto fat bomb snack, *any keto drink	Loaded cauliflower casserole, keto fat bomb snack, *any keto drink	Loaded cauliflower casserole, keto fat bomb snack, *any keto drink	Loaded cauliflower casserole, keto fat bomb snack, *any keto drink	Loaded cauliflower casserole, keto fat bomb snack, *any keto drink	FREESTYLE	FREESTYLE
Snack:	Snack:	Snack:	Snack:	Snack:	Snack:	Snack:
2 keto fat bombs	Great Value snack plate, 3 oz. serving of peanuts and macadamia nuts	Great Value snack plate, 3 oz. serving of peanuts and macadamia nuts	Great Value snack plate, 3 oz. serving of peanuts and macadamia nuts	Great Value snack plate, 3 oz. serving of peanuts and macadamia nuts	2 keto fat bombs	2 keto fat bombs
Cal.: 972	Cal.: 1,203	Cal.: 1,203	Cal.: 1,203	Cal.: 1,203	*Cal.: 416	*Cal.: 616
Carb.: 13.5	Carb.: 17.5	Carb.: 17.5	Carb.: 17.5	Carb.: 17.5	*Carb.: 5.2	*Carb.: 6.2
						*Keep cal. Count

* *Drink your appropriate amount of water! If you're hungry, it's probably because you are actually thirsty. If you choose to drink anything other than water, remember to count your calories and carbs.*

Carbs - Alcohol Sugars - Fiber = Net Carbs

ALL NUTRITIONAL INFORMATION IS APPROXIMATE AND WILL VARY BASED ON ACTUAL INGREDIENTS AND BRANDS USED.

<u>Week 5:</u>

Calories per day: 000–1,500
Carbs per day: 0–20 g

Choose your fasting method and apply it to this plan.

* *Freestyles are you choosing from the list of fast foods that are keto-approved.*

Sunday	Monday	Tuesday	Wednesday	Thursday	Friday	Saturday
Meal 1:	Meal 1:	Meal 1:	Meal 1:	Meal 1:	Meal 1:	Meal 1:
2 boiled eggs, serving of Jimmy Dean fully-cooked pork sausage patties, water to drink	2 boiled eggs, your choice of a cheese stick, water to drink	2 boiled eggs, your choice of a cheese stick, water to drink	2 boiled eggs, your choice of a cheese stick, water to drink	2 boiled eggs, your choice of a cheese stick, water to drink	2 boiled eggs, your choice of a cheese stick, water to drink	2 boiled eggs, serving of Jimmy Dean fully-cooked pork sausage patties, water to drink
Meal 2:	Meal 2:	Meal 2:	Meal 2:	Meal 2:	Meal 2:	Meal 2:
Meatloaf and mashed cauliflower, keto fat bomb snack, *any keto drink	Meatloaf and mashed cauliflower, keto fat bomb snack, *any keto drink	Meatloaf and mashed cauliflower, keto fat bomb snack, *any keto drink	Meatloaf and mashed cauliflower, keto fat bomb snack, *any keto drink	Meatloaf and mashed cauliflower, keto fat bomb snack, *any keto drink	FREESTYLE	FREESTYLE
Snack:	Snack:	Snack:	Snack:	Snack:	Snack:	Snack:
2 keto fat bombs	Serving of pepperoni, Colby jack cheese stick, macadamia nuts	Serving of pepperoni, Colby jack cheese stick, macadamia nuts	Serving of pepperoni, Colby jack cheese stick, macadamia nuts	Serving of pepperoni, Colby jack cheese stick, macadamia nuts	2 keto fat bombs	2 keto fat bombs
Cal.: 980	Cal.: 1,019.9	Cal.: 1,019.9	Cal.: 1,019.9	Cal.: 1,019.9	*Cal.: 416	*Cal.: 616
Carb.: 19.2	Carb.: 16.2	Carb.: 16.2	Carb.: 16.2	Carb.: 16.2	*Carb.: 5.2	*Carb.: 6.2
						*Keep cal. count

* *Drink your appropriate amount of water! If you're hungry, it's probably because you are actually thirsty. If you choose to drink anything other than water, remember to count your calories and carbs.*

Carbs - Alcohol Sugars - Fiber = Net Carbs

ALL NUTRITIONAL INFORMATION IS APPROXIMATE AND WILL VARY BASED ON ACTUAL INGREDIENTS AND BRANDS USED.

Week 6:

Calories per day: 000–1,500
Carbs per day: 0–20 g

Choose your fasting method and apply it to this plan

* *Freestyles are you choosing from the list of fast foods that are keto-approved.*

Sunday	Monday	Tuesday	Wednesday	Thursday	Friday	Saturday
Meal 1:	Meal 1:	Meal 1:	Meal 1:	Meal 1:	Meal 1:	Meal 1:
2 boiled eggs, serving of Jimmy Dean fully-cooked pork sausage patties, water to drink	2 boiled eggs, your choice of a cheese stick, water to drink	2 boiled eggs, your choice of a cheese stick, water to drink	2 boiled eggs, your choice of a cheese stick, water to drink	2 boiled eggs, your choice of a cheese stick, water to drink	2 boiled eggs, your choice of a cheese stick, water to drink	2 boiled eggs, serving of Jimmy Dean fully-cooked pork sausage patties, water to drink
Meal 2:	Meal 2:	Meal 2:	Meal 2:	Meal 2:	Meal 2:	Meal 2:
Cauliflower cheeseburger casserole, keto fat bomb snack, *any keto drink	Cauliflower cheeseburger casserole, keto fat bomb snack, *any keto drink	Cauliflower cheeseburger casserole, keto fat bomb snack, *any keto drink	Cauliflower cheeseburger casserole, keto fat bomb snack, *any keto drink	Cauliflower cheeseburger casserole, keto fat bomb snack, *any keto drink	FREESTYLE	FREESTYLE
Snack:	Snack:	Snack:	Snack:	Snack:	Snack:	Snack:
2 keto fat bombs	Birch Bender's classic yellow cake, serving of peanut butter	Birch Bender's classic yellow cake, serving of peanut butter	Birch Bender's classic yellow cake, serving of peanut butter	Birch Bender's classic yellow cake, serving of peanut butter	2 keto fat bombs	2 keto fat bombs
Cal.: 1,117	Cal.: 1,067	Cal.: 1,067	Cal.: 1,067	Cal.: 1,067	*Cal.: 416	*Cal.: 616
Carb.: 10.8	Carb.: 15.8	Carb.: 15.8	Carb.: 15.8	Carb.: 15.8	*Carb.: 5.2	*Carb.: 6.2
						*Keep cal. count

* *Drink your appropriate amount of water! If you're hungry, it's probably because you are actually thirsty. If you choose to drink anything other than water, remember to count your calories and carbs.*

Carbs - Alcohol Sugars - Fiber = Net Carbs

ALL NUTRITIONAL INFORMATION IS APPROXIMATE AND WILL VARY BASED ON ACTUAL INGREDIENTS AND BRANDS USED.

<u>Week 7:</u>

Calories per day: 000–1,500
Carbs per day: 0–20 g

Choose your fasting method and apply it to this plan.

* *Freestyles are you choosing from the list of fast foods that are keto-approved*

Sunday	Monday	Tuesday	Wednesday	Thursday	Friday	Saturday
Meal 1:	Meal 1:	Meal 1:	Meal 1:	Meal 1:	Meal 1:	Meal 1:
2 boiled eggs, serving of Jimmy Dean fully-cooked pork sausage patties, water to drink	2 boiled eggs, your choice of a cheese stick, water to drink	2 boiled eggs, your choice of a cheese stick, water to drink	2 boiled eggs, your choice of a cheese stick, water to drink	2 boiled eggs, your choice of a cheese stick, water to drink	2 boiled eggs, your choice of a cheese stick, water to drink	2 boiled eggs, serving of Jimmy Dean fully-cooked pork sausage patties, water to drink
Meal 2:	Meal 2:	Meal 2:	Meal 2:	Meal 2:	Meal 2:	Meal 2:
Spaghetti and meatballs, keto fat bomb snack, *any keto drink	Spaghetti and meatballs, keto fat bomb snack, *any keto drink	Spaghetti and meatballs, keto fat bomb snack, *any keto drink	Spaghetti and meatballs, keto fat bomb snack, *any keto drink	Spaghetti and meatballs, keto fat bomb snack, *any keto drink	FREESTYLE	FREESTYLE
Snack:	Snack:	Snack:	Snack:	Snack:	Snack:	Snack:
2 keto fat bombs	Great Value snack plate, 3 oz. keto fat bomb	Great Value snack plate, 3 oz. keto fat bomb	Great Value snack plate, 3 oz. keto fat bomb	Great Value snack plate, 3 oz. keto fat bomb	2 keto fat bombs	2 keto fat bombs
Cal.: 1,061	Cal.: 1,021	Cal.: 1,021	Cal.: 1,021	Cal.: 1,021	*Cal.: 416	*Cal.: 616
Carb.: 14.6	Carb.: 13.6	Carb.: 13.6	Carb.: 13.6	Carb.: 13.6	*Carb.: 5.2	*Carb.: 6.2
						*Keep cal. count

* *Drink your appropriate amount of water! If you're hungry, it's probably because you are actually thirsty. If you choose to drink anything other than water, remember to count your calories and carbs.*

Carbs - Alcohol Sugars - Fiber = Net Carbs

ALL NUTRITIONAL INFORMATION IS APPROXIMATE AND WILL VARY BASED ON ACTUAL INGREDIENTS AND BRANDS USED.

Week 8:

Calories per day: 000–1,500
Carbs per day: 0–20 g

Choose your fasting method and apply it to this plan.

* *Freestyles are you choosing from the list of fast foods that are keto-approved.*

Sunday	Monday	Tuesday	Wednesday	Thursday	Friday	Saturday
Meal 1:	Meal 1:	Meal 1:	Meal 1:	Meal 1:	Meal 1:	Meal 1:
2 boiled eggs, serving of Jimmy Dean fully-cooked pork sausage patties, water to drink	2 boiled eggs, your choice of a cheese stick, water to drink	2 boiled eggs, your choice of a cheese stick, water to drink	2 boiled eggs, your choice of a cheese stick, water to drink	2 boiled eggs, your choice of a cheese stick, water to drink	2 boiled eggs, your choice of a cheese stick, water to drink	2 boiled eggs, serving of Jimmy Dean fully-cooked pork sausage patties, water to drink
Meal 2:	Meal 2:	Meal 2:	Meal 2:	Meal 2:	Meal 2:	Meal 2:
Jalapeño beef casserole, keto fat bomb snack, *any keto drink	Jalapeño beef casserole, keto fat bomb snack, *any keto drink	Jalapeño beef casserole, keto fat bomb snack, *any keto drink	Jalapeño beef casserole, keto fat bomb snack, *any keto drink	Jalapeño beef casserole, keto fat bomb snack, *any keto drink	FREESTYLE	FREESTYLE
Snack:	Snack:	Snack:	Snack:	Snack:	Snack:	Snack:
2 keto fat bombs	Serving of pork rinds, Colby jack cheese stick, serving of olives, serving of peperoni	Serving of pork rinds, Colby jack cheese stick, serving of olives, serving of peperoni	Serving of pork rinds, Colby jack cheese stick, serving of olives, serving of peperoni	Serving of pork rinds, Colby jack cheese stick, serving of olives, serving of peperoni	2 keto fat bombs	2 keto fat bombs
Cal.: 1,281	Cal.: 1,260.9	Cal.: 1,260.9	Cal.: 1,260.9	Cal.: 1,260.9	*Cal.: 416	*Cal.: 616
Carb.: 10.2	Carb.: 5.2	Carb.: 5.2	Carb.: 5.2	Carb.: 5.2	*Carb.: 5.2	*Carb.: 6.2
						*Keep cal. count

* *Drink your appropriate amount of water! If you're hungry, it's probably because you are actually thirsty. If you choose to drink anything other than water, remember to count your calories and carbs.*

Carbs - Alcohol Sugars - Fiber = Net Carbs

ALL NUTRITIONAL INFORMATION IS APPROXIMATE AND WILL VARY BASED ON ACTUAL INGREDIENTS AND BRANDS USED.

Week 9:

Calories per day: 000–1,500
Carbs per day: 0–20 g

Choose your fasting method and apply it to this plan.

* *Freestyles are you choosing from the list of fast foods that are keto-approved.*

Sunday	Monday	Tuesday	Wednesday	Thursday	Friday	Saturday
Meal 1:	Meal 1:	Meal 1:	Meal 1:	Meal 1:	Meal 1:	Meal 1:
2 boiled eggs, serving of Jimmy Dean fully-cooked pork sausage patties, water to drink	2 boiled eggs, your choice of a cheese stick, water to drink	2 boiled eggs, your choice of a cheese stick, water to drink	2 boiled eggs, your choice of a cheese stick, water to drink	2 boiled eggs, your choice of a cheese stick, water to drink	2 boiled eggs, your choice of a cheese stick, water to drink	2 boiled eggs, serving of Jimmy Dean fully-cooked pork sausage patties, water to drink
Meal 2:	Meal 2:	Meal 2:	Meal 2:	Meal 2:	Meal 2:	Meal 2:
Club lettuce wrap, keto fat bomb snack, *any keto drink	Club lettuce wrap, keto fat bomb snack, *any keto drink	Club lettuce wrap, keto fat bomb snack, *any keto drink	Club lettuce wrap, keto fat bomb snack, *any keto drink	Club lettuce wrap, keto fat bomb snack, *any keto drink	FREESTYLE	FREESTYLE
Snack:	Snack:	Snack:	Snack:	Snack:	Snack:	Snack:
2 keto fat bombs	Great Value snack plate, 3 oz. serving of peanuts	Great Value snack plate, 3 oz. serving of peanuts	Great Value snack plate, 3 oz. serving of peanuts	Great Value snack plate, 3 oz. serving of peanuts	2 keto fat bombs	2 keto fat bombs
Cal.: 1,211	Cal.: 1,242	Cal.: 1,242	Cal.: 1,242	Cal.: 1,242	*Cal.: 416	*Cal.: 616
Carb.: 12.1	Carb.: 13.1	Carb.: 13.1	Carb.: 13.1	Carb.: 13.1	*Carb.: 5.2	*Carb.: 6.2
						*Keep cal. count

* *Drink your appropriate amount of water! If you're hungry, it's probably because you are actually thirsty. If you choose to drink anything other than water, remember to count your calories and carbs.*

Carbs - Alcohol Sugars - Fiber = Net Carbs

ALL NUTRITIONAL INFORMATION IS APPROXIMATE AND WILL VARY BASED ON ACTUAL INGREDIENTS AND BRANDS USED.

Week 10:

Calories per day: 000–1,500

Carbs per day: 0–20 g

Choose your fasting method and apply it to this plan.

* *Freestyles are you choosing from the list of fast foods that are keto-approved.*

Sunday	Monday	Tuesday	Wednesday	Thursday	Friday	Saturday
Meal 1:	Meal 1:	Meal 1:	Meal 1:	Meal 1:	Meal 1:	Meal 1:
2 boiled eggs, serving of Jimmy Dean fully-cooked pork sausage patties, water to drink	2 boiled eggs, your choice of a cheese stick, water to drink	2 boiled eggs, your choice of a cheese stick, water to drink	2 boiled eggs, your choice of a cheese stick, water to drink	2 boiled eggs, your choice of a cheese stick, water to drink	2 boiled eggs, your choice of a cheese stick, water to drink	2 boiled eggs, serving of Jimmy Dean fully-cooked pork sausage patties, water to drink
Meal 2:	Meal 2:	Meal 2:	Meal 2:	Meal 2:	Meal 2:	Meal 2:
Chicken salad, keto fat bomb snack, *any keto drink	Chicken salad, keto fat bomb snack, *any keto drink	Chicken salad, keto fat bomb snack, *any keto drink	Chicken salad, keto fat bomb snack, *any keto drink	Chicken salad, keto fat bomb snack, *any keto drink	FREESTYLE	FREESTYLE
Snack:	Snack:	Snack:	Snack:	Snack:	Snack:	Snack:
2 keto fat bombs	Great Value snack plate, 3 oz. keto fat bomb	Great Value snack plate, 3 oz. keto fat bomb	Great Value snack plate, 3 oz. keto fat bomb	Great Value snack plate, 3 oz. keto fat bomb	2 keto fat bomb	2 keto fat bombs
Cal.: 1,027	Cal.: 987	Cal.: 987	Cal.: 987	Cal.: 987	*Cal.: 416	*Cal.: 616
Carb.: 10.2	Carb.: 9.2	Carb.: 9.2	Carb.: 9.2	Carb.: 9.2	*Carb.: 5.2	*Carb.: 6.2
						*Keep cal. count

* *Drink your appropriate amount of water! If you're hungry, it's probably because you are actually thirsty. If you choose to drink anything other than water, remember to count your calories and carbs.*

Carbs - Alcohol Sugars - Fiber = Net Carbs

ALL NUTRITIONAL INFORMATION IS APPROXIMATE AND WILL VARY BASED ON ACTUAL INGREDIENTS AND BRANDS USED.

Food and Activity Log

Date: Monday, 00/00/00

Time:	Food and Drink	Thoughts/Feelings	Am I Hungry?
8:00 a.m.	2 boiled eggs, Colby jack cheese stick, water	I'm late for work, let me place these eggs and cheese in a bag.	No
12:00 p.m.	Spaghetti and meatballs, water, Perrier Water	I'm so glad to be taking this break!	Yes
3:00 p.m.	Keto fat bomb, water	When am I going home? I'm so sleepy! Feeling meh.	Not really
5:00 p.m.	Snack plate, water	Yes, home at last!	Somewhat
8:00 p.m.	Keto fat bomb, water, Perrier Water	I'm bored, what can I do?	No

Food for thought: Think about what you did to be active between your meals today, what did you personally do for yourself today, what time is the perfect cutoff eating time for your schedule. Was there anything about the day that made you feel good? Are you eating because you are bored?

Food and Activity Log

Date: _______________________________

Time:	Food and Drink	Thoughts/Feelings	Am I Hungry?	Fast

During my keto journey, I did the elliptical for 45 minutes on weekends (Saturday and Sunday).

I believe it will be very beneficial to your muscles, skin, and entire body if you get it active.

You are helping it get used to the fat that you are losing.

Time:	Physical Activity:

Food and Activity Log

Date: _______________________________

Time:	Food and Drink	Thoughts/Feelings	Am I Hungry?	Fast

During my keto journey, I did the elliptical for 45 minutes on weekends (Saturday and Sunday).

I believe it will be very beneficial to your muscles, skin, and entire body if you get it active.

You are helping it get used to the fat that you are losing.

Time:	Physical Activity:

Food and Activity Log

Date: _______________________________

Time:	Food and Drink	Thoughts/Feelings	Am I Hungry?	Fast

During my keto journey, I did the elliptical for 45 minutes on weekends (Saturday and Sunday).

I believe it will be very beneficial to your muscles, skin, and entire body if you get it active.

You are helping it get used to the fat that you are losing.

Time:	Physical Activity:

Food and Activity Log

Date: _______________________________

Time:	Food and Drink	Thoughts/Feelings	Am I Hungry?	Fast

During my keto journey, I did the elliptical for 45 minutes on weekends (Saturday and Sunday).

I believe it will be very beneficial to your muscles, skin, and entire body if you get it active.

You are helping it get used to the fat that you are losing.

Time:	Physical Activity:

Food and Activity Log

Date: _______________________

Time:	Food and Drink	Thoughts/Feelings	Am I Hungry?	Fast

During my keto journey, I did the elliptical for 45 minutes on weekends (Saturday and Sunday).

I believe it will be very beneficial to your muscles, skin, and entire body if you get it active.

You are helping it get used to the fat that you are losing.

Time:	Physical Activity:

Food and Activity Log

Date: _______________________________

Time:	Food and Drink	Thoughts/Feelings	Am I Hungry?	Fast

During my keto journey, I did the elliptical for 45 minutes on weekend (Saturday and Sunday).

I believe it will be very beneficial to your muscles, skin, and entire body if you get it active.

You are helping it get used to the fat that you are losing.

Time:	Physical Activity:

Food and Activity Log

Date: ___________________________

Time:	Food and Drink	Thoughts/Feelings	Am I Hungry?	Fast

During my keto journey, I did the elliptical for 45 minutes on weekends (Saturday and Sunday).

I believe it will be very beneficial to your muscles, skin, and entire body if you get it active.

You are helping it get used to the fat that you are losing.

Time:	Physical Activity:

The Woes of Keto . . .

There is always a bad side to everything—keto is not exempt.

As I've said before, my keto experience will without a doubt be different from your keto experience. There are changes—some big, some small—that your body will go through while in ketosis. I believe that monitoring your body weekly is crucial. This is not to scare you.

Remember that we are fighting with ourselves, not against.

Monitoring your body will allow you to notice the small things that will help you in the long run. Monitoring your body also means frequently weighing yourself.

My skin tone is a darker complexion. I noticed that I had developed a rash that led from the front part of my upper arms to my back. I'm not sure when I developed it, but naturally, I became cautious of everything. I thought that it was from my Dove body wash, then maybe my Daisy perfume, then perhaps my laundry detergent.

I did some research and found out that the rash is very common for those on the keto diet.

The rash is called prurigo pigmentosa. The rash typically appears on the upper parts of the body, rarely the face. They appear as red (black in my case) itchy, inflamed patches. The cause of the rash is unknown, but it has been reported from those that are on the keto diet.

I began to treat the rash as if it was eczema, and it began to fade. I, however, still insist that you consult your physician about the matter. I used Eucerin cream, but it may not work as well for you.

Remember, I'm not a doctor, I dropped out of phlebotomy school.

Another thing to monitor is your bowel movements. Your poop! You will become constipated, and you will get diarrhea.

The best that I can tell you is to drink lots of water, eat broccoli (it contains sulforaphane, which protects the gut and eases digestion), avocados, and berries (black berries and raspberries are rich in fiber). Olive oil! I almost forgot that olive oil also has a mild laxative effect as well.

Those who are able to have a menstrual cycle, monitor it!

I found that being on the keto diet helped stabilize my cycle. It was totally predictable (except for that one time, but that doesn't count because . . . well, mind your business, not mine, thanks!).

You want to make sure nothing out of the norm is going on with your cycle. I have read articles from Well Versed and Everydayhealth.com that mentions a double cycle in a month. That has happened to me while on keto. However, they were both short, lasting only 2–3 days long.

Other articles mention reports of no cycles at all.

Your cycle may become long or longer than your usual.

While on my cycle, I also noticed the development of an insatiable appetite. I didn't experience the want for more food every cycle, but when I did, it was honestly the worst. This urge to eat always happened around 3:00 p.m., and I could never get enough food!

Watch out for this. Luckily, I never gained any weight from it. It simply seemed that my body needed more calories, protein, fiber, something! I'm not sure why I experienced that, but I did want to give a heads up on it.

Bottom line, monitor your cycle, folks.

Something else that I was not aware of was the amount of camps that you would get! I did not know that you could get cramps in your toes. The first time it happened to me, I almost called off of work. Seriously!

I got cramps in some of the oddest places! I cried and prayed, mostly because I'm dramatic.

I started to drink more water to help with this, and it helped some. I stopped receiving the cramps as much, but I still got them frequently.

This, fortunately, did not happen to me, but there are cases of severe bad breath while on the keto diet. I'm not sure as to why people have experienced this, but do watch out for this, and do take in your fair share of water every day.

Wrapping It All Up

Thanks to Kanye's workout plan—

Just kidding! Losing weight on the keto diet does give you all the vibes from that song though.

At least for me it does.

In all seriousness, I appreciate you, my fellow keto dieter.

I appreciate you for taking the time to create a routine that will better your life.

I appreciate you for having the courage to admit that there is something toxic in your life, be it a food relationship, work-related, family-centered, etc.

I appreciate your drive for better self-control.

I appreciate you for finding the courage to start a workout routine.

I know how intimidating the gym can seem!

I appreciate you for taking a chance on yourself.

I appreciate you for wanting to find new ways to love your body and life.

I appreciate you for finding your perfect fasting method, if any at all!

I appreciate you for not stopping when you plateaued, and you will!

I appreciate the curiosity that lies within you, the curiosity that prompted you to purchase my book and explore it—my book of all books.

I appreciate you for trusting my knowledge enough to help you through this new thing that we call a keto diet.

Thank you!

Excellent Resources for Recipes

https://thebigmansworld.com
https://thebestketorecipes.com
https://www.eatwell101.com
https://www.delish.com
https://www.smalltownwoman.com
https://gypsyplate.com
https://www.eatyourselfskinny.com
https://mylifecookbook.com
https://realsimplegood.com

During my keto journey, I have used all these listed sites for my keto meals and snacks.

The Big Man's World has the best recipe for keto peanut butter cookies in my opinion. Delish, of course, is the cheat code for all your favorite normal meals. I'm a huge fan of fried pork chops, and I found a great recipe for pork chops and mashed cauliflower on their site.

Whenever you have time, or are in the midst of grocery shopping, pop in on any of these sites and get some recipe ideas. The great majority of these recipes are very simple, and you can make small adjustments to your liking. One recipe insisted on adding Worcestershire sauce and Dijon to my cheeseburger casserole, and I omitted it! It sounded gross).

Whether you think you can,
or think you can't, you're right.

—Henry Ford

10 months on keto diet, 130 pounds down

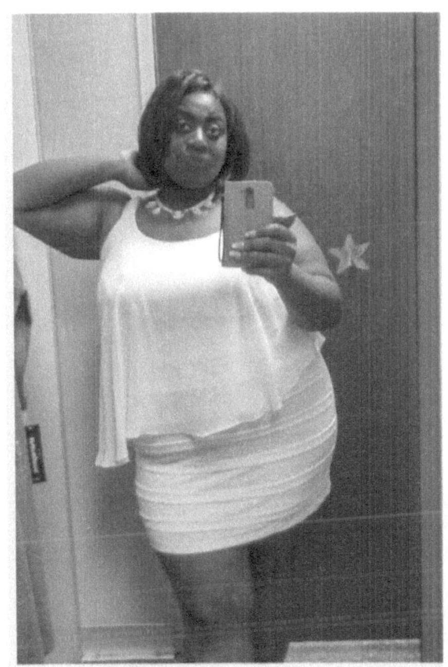

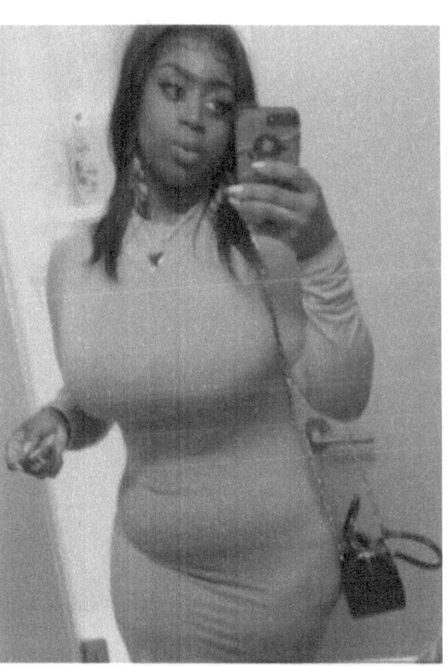